The Keto Diet Breakfast Cookbook for Women Over 50

Super Delicious and Super Easy Recipes to Burn Fat

Katie Attanasio

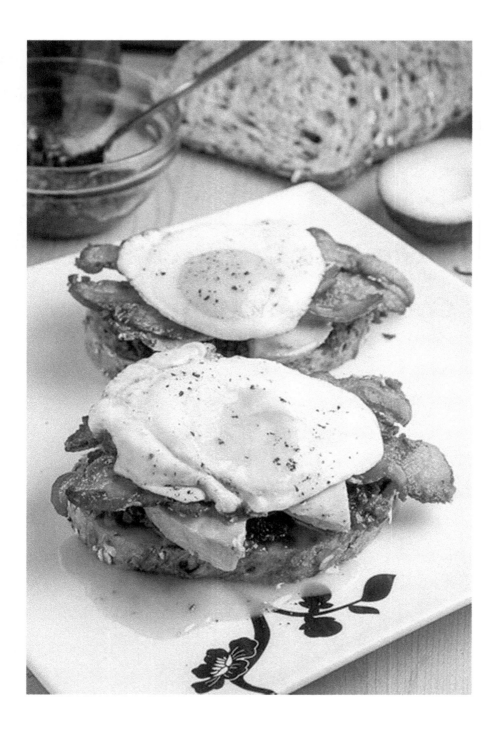

a result of the use of information contained within this document, including, but not limited to, — errors, omissions, or inaccuracies.

Table of Contents

50 Keto Breakfast Recipes 8

1   Keto Italian Breakfast Casserole 8

2   Keto Salmon-Filled Avocados 11

3   Keto Croque Madame 12

4   Keto Salami And Brie Cheese Plate 15

5   Keto Mackerel And Egg Plate 16

6   Keto Turkey Plate 17

7   Keto Cauliflower Hash With Eggs And Poblano Peppers 19

8   Keto Seafood Omelet 21

9   Keto Rutabaga Patties With Smoked Salmon 23

10   Keto Rutabaga Fritters With Bacon 25

11   Keto Coconut Pancakes 27

12   Keto Porridge 29

13   Keto Western Omelet 30

14   Keto Breakfast Tapas 32

15   Keto Scrambled Eggs With Halloumi Cheese 33

16   Prawn And Herb Omelet 35

17   Pumpkin Spice Overnight Oats 38

18   Keto Breakfast Grits 40

19   Keto Mushroom Sausage Skillet 42

20   Keto Lemon Donut Holes 44

21   Keto Eggs Benedict 46

22   Huevos Rancheros 49

23   Keto Breakfast Enchiladas 51

24   Keto Southern Shakshuka 53

25   Keto Chicken and Waffle Sandwiches 55

26   Keto Pepperoni Pizza Quiche 58

27   Keto Blueberry Pancake Bites 60

28   Gooey Keto Cinnamon Rolls 62

29   Berry Coconut Oatmeal 65

30   Keto Breakfast Bowl 67

31   Asparagus and Gruyere Keto Quiche 69

32   Keto Lemon Sugar Poppy Seed Scones 71

33   Eggs Benedict Casserole 73

34   Bacon Kale and Tomato Frittata 75

35   Caprese Egg Casserole 77

36   Keto Sausage Gravy and Biscuit Bake 79

37   Mini Pizza Egg Bakes 81

38   Instant Pot Crustless Quiche Lorraine 83

39   Vegetarian Three Cheese Quiche Stuffed Peppers 85

40   No-tatoes Bubble 'n' Squeak 87

41   Bacon Breakfast Bagels 89

42   Spinach, Herb & Feta Wrap 91

43   Salmon Benny Breakfast Bombs 93

44   Ham, Ricotta, and Spinach Casserole 95

45   Keto Zucchini Bread with Walnuts 97

46   Lemon Raspberry Sweet Rolls 99

47   Keto Faux Sous Vide Egg Bites 102

48   Savory Sage and Cheddar Waffles 104

49   Keto Lemon Poppyseed Muffins 106

50   Low Carb Mock McGriddle Casserole 108

50 Keto Breakfast Recipes

1   Keto Italian Breakfast Casserole

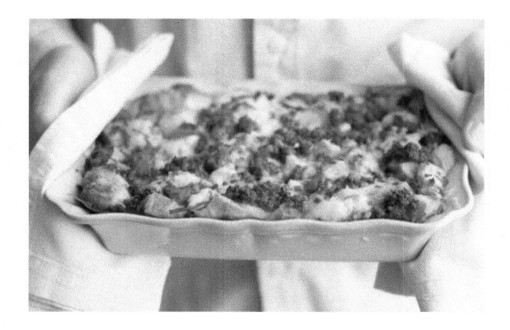

Servings: 4 | **Time:** 1 hr. | **Difficulty:** Easy

Nutrients per serving: Calories: 801 kcal | Fat: 71g | Carbohydrates: 7g | Protein: 16g | Fiber: 1g

Ingredients

8 Eggs

1 Cup Cheddar Cheese, Shredded

1/4 Cup Butter

1/4 Cup Basil, Fresh & Chopped

Salt, To Taste

3/4 Cup Cauliflower, Chopped

1 Cup Heavy Whipping Cream

Black Pepper, To Taste

1 & 1/2 Cups Italian Sausage, Fresh

Method

1.   Preheat the oven to 375 degrees F.

2.   Heat the butter in a pan over medium-high heat until it melts and sauté the cauliflower in it. When it get softer, take out and set aside.

3.   Then sauté the sausage in the same pan by breaking it into crumbs with the spoon and add the salt and pepper in it. Cook it thoroughly.

4.   Whisk the eggs, cheese, cream, salt and pepper together in a bowl until smooth. Set aside.

5.   Brush a baking dish (8x8 inches) with oil or butter and put the sautéed cauliflower and sausage in it. Pour the egg mixture on it and top with basil.

6.   Put the baking dish in the preheated oven and bake the casserole until becomes golden brown, for about 30–40 minutes.

7.   Take out once all set and cooked and serve.

2   Keto Salmon-Filled Avocados

Servings: 2 | **Time**: 10 mins | **Difficulty:** Beginner

Nutrients per serving: Calories: 715 kcal | Fat: 64g | Carbohydrates: 6g | Protein: 22g | Fiber: 13g

Ingredients

3/4 Cup Sour Cream

Black Pepper, To Taste

3/4 Cup Salmon, Smoked

Salt, To Taste

2 Avocados, Halved & Pitted

2 Tbsps. Lemon Juice (Optional)

Method

1.   Take the halved and pitted avocados and fill their hole with a dollop of sour cream and top with smoked salmon.

2.   Sprinkle the salt and pepper on top and drizzle the lemon juice if desired.

3   Keto Croque Madame

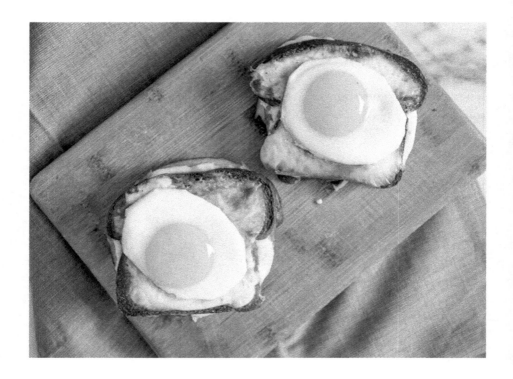

Servings: 2 | **Time**: 25 mins | **Difficulty:** Medium

Nutrients per serving: Calories: 1218 kcal | Fat: 105g | Carbohydrates: 10g | Protein: 58g | Fiber: 5g

Ingredients

1 Cup Cottage Cheese

4 Eggs

3 Tsps. Psyllium Husk Powder, Ground

4 Tbsps. Butter

2/3 Cup Smoked Deli Ham

1/4 Cup Cheddar Cheese, Sliced

2 Tbsps. Red Onion, Chopped Finely

Serving:

2 Eggs

2 Tbsps. Butter

1 1/2 Cups Baby Spinach

4 Tbsps. Olive Oil

1/2 Tbsp. Red Wine Vinegar

Salt, To Taste

Black Pepper, To Taste

Method

1. Combine the eggs, cottage cheese, psyllium husk powder in a bowl and whisk them well, until a smooth batter is formed. Set aside for five minutes to let it thicken.

2.   Melt the butter in a frying pan over medium flame and put the spoonful batter in it to make pancakes. Cook the pancakes on both sides until become golden brown.

3.   Put the sliced ham, onion, and cheddar cheese on one pancake and put the other on top, to make a sandwich.

4.   Combine the vinegar, spinach, oil, salt, and pepper in a bowl to make the vinaigrette.

5.   Make fried eggs with the remaining butter and put them on top of the sandwiches.

6.   Serve the warm Croque Madame with spinach vinaigrette.

4   Keto Salami And Brie Cheese Plate

Servings: 2 | **Time:** 5 mins | **Difficulty:** Beginner

Nutrients per serving: Calories: 1218 kcal | Fat: 115g | Carbohydrates: 5g | Protein: 39g | Fiber: 10g

Ingredients

3/4 Cup Brie Cheese

1/2 Cup Salami

1 & 1/2 Cups Lettuce

1 Avocado

5 Tbsps. Macadamia Nuts

1/4 Cup Olive Oil

Method

1.   Combine all the ingredients in a salad bowl and toss well.

2.   Serve and enjoy.

5   Keto Mackerel And Egg Plate

Servings: 2 | **Time:** 15 mins | **Difficulty**: Beginner

Nutrients per serving: Calories: 689 kcal | Fat: 59g | Carbohydrates: 4g | Protein: 35g | Fiber: 1g

Ingredients

1/4 Cup Olive Oil

Black Pepper, To Taste

1/4 Cup Red Onion, Sliced

1 Cup Mackerel In Tomato Sauce, Canned

1 & 1/2 Cups Lettuce

Salt, To Taste

4 Eggs

2 Tbsps. Butter

Method

1.   Melt the butter in a frying pan and fry the eggs according to your preference. Dish it out on a serving plate.

2.   Put the onion slices, lettuce, and mackerel on the plate beside eggs. Sprinkle salt and pepper on it and drizzle the olive oil on the salad. Serve and enjoy.

6   Keto Turkey Plate

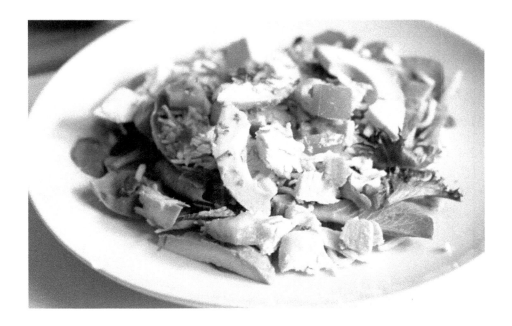

Servings: 2 | **Time**: 8 mins | **Difficulty:** Easy

Nutrients per serving: Calories: 660 kcal | Fat: 60g | Carbohydrates: 7g | Protein: 13g | Fiber: 7g

Ingredients

1/4 Cup Olive Oil

1/3 Cup Cream Cheese

Salt, To Taste

1 & 1/2 Cups Lettuce

Black Pepper, To Taste

3/4 Cup Deli Turkey

1 Avocado, Sliced

Method

1.   Combine all the ingredients in a bowl and toss well.

2.   Divide it into two servings.

7   Keto Cauliflower Hash With Eggs And Poblano Peppers

Servings: 2 | **Time:** 25 mins | **Difficulty**: Easy

Nutrients per serving: Calories: 897 kcal | Fat: 87g | Carbohydrates: 9g | Protein: 17g | Fiber: 6g

Ingredients

4 Eggs

Black Pepper, To Taste

1 Tsp. Olive Oil

2 Cups Cauliflower, Grated

Salt, To Taste

1/2 Cup Mayonnaise

6 Tbsps. Butter

1/3 Cup Poblano Peppers

1 Tsp. Garlic Powder

Method

1.   Melt the butter in a pan and sauté the grated cauliflower in it. Sprinkle with salt and pepper and stir to combine. Take out once fried and set aside.

2.   Stir fry the poblano peppers in the same pan in melted butter. Once their skin starts to bubble, take off the heat and set aside.

3.   Whisk mayonnaise and garlic powder in a bowl and set aside.

4.   Fry the eggs in the butter according to your preference and sprinkle the salt and pepper on them.

5.   Serve the fried eggs with the sautéed poblanos and cauliflower hash. Put a dollop of the seasoned mayo on top.

8   Keto Seafood Omelet

Servings: 2 | **Time:** 20 mins | **Difficulty**: Easy

Nutrients per serving: Calories: 870 kcal | Fat: 82g | Carbohydrates: 4g | Protein: 27g | Fiber: 1g

Ingredients

6 Eggs

4 Tbsps. Olive Oil

Salt, To Taste

2/3 Cup Shrimp, Cooked

1 Red Chili Pepper

Black Pepper, To Taste

1/2 Tsp. Cumin, Ground

1 Tbsp. Chives, Fresh

1/2 Cup Mayonnaise

2 Garlic Cloves, Minced (Optional)

Method

1.   Preheat a broiler.

2.   Combine the shrimps with 2 tbsps. olive oil, garlic, red chili, ground cumin, salt, and pepper in a bowl. Mix them well and put the marinated shrimps in the broiler.

3.   Once the shrimps cooked through, take out of the broiler, and let cool.

4.   When cooled, add in the chives and mayo to the shrimps.

5.   Whisk the eggs with salt and pepper in a bowl and fry the omelet in the remaining olive oil in a non- stick pan.

6.   When the omelet is half cooked, add in the shrimp mixture and fold. Cooke at low heat and once the eggs are set dish out and serve hot.

9   Keto Rutabaga Patties With Smoked Salmon

Servings: 2 | **Time:** 30 mins | **Difficulty:** Medium

Nutrients per serving: Calories: 660 kcal | Fat: 60g | Carbohydrates: 7g | Protein: 13g | Fiber: 7g

Ingredients

Rutabaga patties:

1/2 Cup Butter

1/2 Tsp. Onion Powder

1/4 Tsp. Pepper

3 Tbsps. Coconut Flour

1 Tsp. Salt

1 & 1/2 Cups Rutabaga, Peeled & Grated

4 Eggs

1 Cup. Halloumi Cheese, Shredded

1/8 Cup Turmeric (Optional)

For Serving:

2 & 1/2 Cups Leafy Greens

1 & 1/4 Cups Salmon, Smoked

2 Tbsps. Lemon Juice

1 Cup Mayonnaise

Method

1.   Combine all the patties ingredients in a bowl except butter and mix well. Let it rest for a few minutes.

2.   Melt the butter in a skillet and put the spoonful of rutabaga mixture in it to make 12 patties out of it. Fry the patties over medium heat.

3.   Cook on both sides for a few minutes and dish out once golden brown.

4.   Serve with the smoked salmon, a dollop of mayonnaise, green salad with a little lemon juice squeezed on it.

10   Keto Rutabaga Fritters With Bacon

Servings: 4 | **Time:** 30 mins | **Difficulty**: Medium

Nutrients per serving: Calories: 955 kcal | Fat: 89g | Carbohydrates: 10g | Protein: 24g | Fiber: 6g

Ingredients

Rutabaga Fritters:

3 Tbsps. Coconut Flour

2 Cups Rutabaga, Peeled & Grated

1/2 Tsp. Onion Powder

1/3 Cup Butter

3/4 Cup Halloumi Cheese, Shredded

1/4 Tsp. Pepper

4 Eggs

1 Tsp. Salt

1/8 Tsp. Turmeric

For Serving:

2 & 1/2 Cups Leafy Greens

1 Cup Mayonnaise

3/4 Cup Bacon

Method

1.   Combine all the fritters ingredients in a bowl except butter and mix well. Let it rest for a few minutes.

2.   Melt the butter in a skillet and put the spoonful of rutabaga mixture in it to make 12 fritters out of it. Fry them over medium heat.

3.   Cook on both sides for a few minutes and dish out once golden brown.

4.   Serve with mayonnaise, crispy bacon, and green salad.

11   Keto Coconut Pancakes

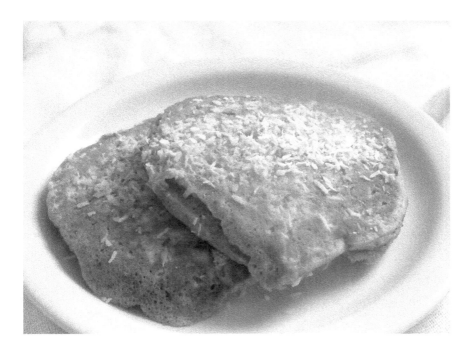

Servings: 4 | **Time:** 40 mins | **Difficulty:** Medium

Nutrients per serving: Calories: 279 kcal | Fat: 24g | Carbohydrates: 3g | Protein: 11g | Fiber: 6g

Ingredients

3/4 Cup Coconut Milk

6 Eggs

2 Tbsps. Coconut Oil, Melted

1/8 Tsp. Salt

1 Tsp. Baking Powder Butter, For Frying

1/2 Cup Coconut Flour

Method

1.   Combine all the ingredients, except butter, in a bowl and whisk or beat them well, until a smooth batter is formed, without lumps.

2.   Heat the butter in a pan, until it melts and put a spoonful of batter on it and spread it with the back of spoon evenly. Flip once done from one side and cook both sides until become golden. Similarly fry the pancakes for the remaining batter at low or medium heat.

12   Keto Porridge

Servings: 1 | **Time**: 10 mins | **Difficulty**: Easy

Nutrients per serving: Calories: 644 kcal | Fat: 64g | Carbohydrates: 5g | Protein: 12g | Fiber: 5g

Ingredients

1 Tbsp. Chia Seeds

1 Tbsp. Sesame Seeds

1 Egg

1/3 Cup Heavy Whipping Cream

1/8 Tsp. Salt

2 Tbsps. Coconut Oil

Method

1.   Combine all the ingredients, except butter, in a bowl and mix well until a smooth mixture is formed. Let it rest for 2–3 minutes.

2.   Meanwhile, heat the coconut oil in a pan on medium.

3.   Pour in the egg and creamy mixture in the oil and stir well. Let it simmer until your desired consistency and thickness is attained but do not boil it.

4.   Transfer to a serving bowl, once done and serve hot.

13   Keto Western Omelet

Servings: 2 | **Time:** 30 mins | **Difficulty:** Easy

Nutrients per serving: Calories: 708 kcal | Fat: 58g | Carbohydrates: 6g | Protein: 40g | Fiber: 1g

Ingredients

2/3 Cup Deli Ham, Smoked & Diced

6 Eggs

Salt, To Taste

3/4 Cup Cheddar Cheese, Shredded

1/2 Onion, Chopped Finely

Black Pepper, To Taste

2 Tbsps. Heavy Whipping Cream

1/2 Green Bell Pepper, Chopped Finely

4 Tbsps. Butter

Method

1.   Combine the eggs with whipping cream, half of the cheddar cheese, salt and pepper and whisk until the mixture becomes creamy and fluffy.

2.   Heat the butter in a frying pan over medium flame until it melts and sauté the onion, peppers, and diced ham in it for a few minutes until they become soft.

3.   Add in the egg mixture and cook the omelet over reduced heat to avoid the burning of egg. Once the eggs are set, sprinkle the remaining cheddar cheese on it.

4.   Once the cheese melts, transfer the omelet to a serving dish and enjoy.

14   Keto Breakfast Tapas

Servings: 4 | **Time:** 15 mins | **Difficulty:** Easy

Nutrients per serving: Calories: 573 kcal | Fat: 50g | Carbohydrates: 6g | Protein: 24g | Fiber: 1g

Ingredients

1 Cup Chorizo, Diced

1/2 Cup Cucumber, Diced

1 Cup Cheddar Cheese, Shredded

1/2 Cup Mayonnaise

1/4 Cup Red Bell Peppers, Diced

1 Cup Prosciutto, Sliced

Method

1.   Combine all the ingredients in a bowl and toss well to mix.

2.   Divide into four servings and enjoy.

15   Keto Scrambled Eggs With Halloumi Cheese

Servings: 2 | **Time:** 20 mins | **Difficulty:** Easy

Nutrients per serving: Calories: 647 kcal | Fat: 57g | Carbohydrates: 4g | Protein: 28g | Fiber: 1g

Ingredients

2 Tbsps. Olive Oil

Salt, To Taste

4 Eggs

4 Tbsps. Parsley, Fresh & Chopped Black

Pepper, To Taste

1/3 Cup Halloumi Cheese, Diced

7 Tbsps. Olives, Pitted

1/3 Cup Bacon, Diced

2 Scallions, Chopped

Method

1.   Combine the eggs, parsley, salt, and pepper in a bowl and whisk well to form a smooth mixture. Set aside.

2.   Take a frying pan and heat the olive oil in it over medium-high flame.

3.   Sauté the scallions, bacon, and halloumi cheese in it until they become golden brown. Then add in the egg mixture and lower the flame.

4.   Cook the eggs for a while and add in the olives.

5.   Stir for a few of minutes, transfer to a serving plate once done.

16   Prawn And Herb Omelet

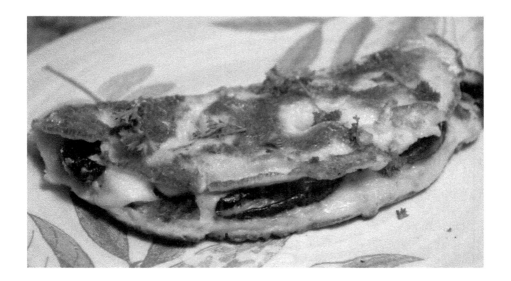

Servings: 4 | **Time:** 25 mins | **Difficulty:** Easy

Nutrients per serving: Calories: 599 kcal | Fat: 15g | Carbohydrates: 11g | Protein: 45g

Ingredients

1 & 1/2 Cups Prawns, Cooked & Chopped

14 Eggs

Nori Sheets, Toasted & Cut Into Squares

1 Cup Milk

Sesame Seeds, Toasted

1/2 Cup Dill, Chopped

2 Spring Onions, Sliced

1/2 Cup Parsley, Chopped

1/4 Cup Butter, Diced

1/2 Cup Chives, Chopped

1 Cucumber, Sliced

1 Fennel, Sliced

Salt, To Taste

Black Pepper, To Taste

Lemon-Tahini Dressing

2 Tbsps. Chives, Chopped

1 Tbsp. Tahini

2 Tbsps. Extra Virgin Olive Oil

2 Tsps. Honey

2 Tbsps. Lemon

1 Tbsp. Water

Method

1.   Combine all the ingredients of lemon tahini dressing in a bowl and mix well.

2.   Put the eggs, milk, parsley, chives, and dill in a bowl and whisk them.

3.   Put half the butter in a frying pan and heat it over medium-high heat.

4.   Once melted, pour half the egg mixture in it, and swirl the pan to spread in the pan. After a minute when the eggs are half cooked, add half the cooked shrimps in it and fold gently.

5.   Season with salt and pepper and cook for a minute or two until eggs are set and the prawns are warm. Transfer to a serving dish.

6.   Repeat this with other half of butter, egg mixture and prawns.

7.   Put the sliced spring onions, cucumber nori and sesame seeds on top of the omelet and serve with the tahini dressing.

17   Pumpkin Spice Overnight Oats

Servings: 2 | **Time**: 8 hrs. | **Difficulty**: Easy

Nutrients per serving: Calories: 444 kcal | Fat: 41.3g | Carbohydrates: 5.1g | Protein: 15.4g

Ingredients

2 Tbsps. Coconut Milk, Unsweetened

1/2 Cup Hemp Hearts

1 Tbsp. MCT Oil

1/3 Cup Coconut Milk, From Carton

3/4 Tsp. Pumpkin Pie Spice

1/3 Cup Coffee, Brewed

2 Tbsps. Pecans, Chopped

2 Tbsps. Pumpkin Puree

1 Tbsp. Chia Seeds

1/4 Tsp. Cinnamon, Ground

2 Tsps. Erythritol, Powdered

Sea Salt, To Taste

1/2 Tsp. Vanilla Extract

Method

1.	Combine all the ingredients except carton coconut milk, cinnamon, and pecans in a bowl and mix well.

2.	Transfer to a mason jar with a lid and refrigerate overnight.

3.	Add in the carton coconut milk and mix well.

4.	Sprinkle the chopped pecans and cinnamon powder on top.

18   Keto Breakfast Grits

Servings: 2 | **Time:** 15 mins | **Difficulty**: Easy

Nutrients per serving: Calories: 484 kcal | Fat: 43.1g | Carbohydrates: 8.1g | Protein: 17.8g

Ingredients

1/4 Cup Cheddar Cheese

1/4 Tsp. Garlic Powder

2 Tbsps. Butter

1/4 Cup Hemp Hearts

2 Cups Cauliflower Rice

1/4 Cup Heavy Cream

1/2 Cup Cremini Mushrooms

1 Cup Almond Milk

Salt, To Taste

Black Pepper, To Taste

Method

1.　　Heat half the butter in a pan and sauté the mushrooms in it for 2-3 minutes over medium heat. Sprinkle some salt and pepper in it and take off the heat once become softer. Set aside.

2.　　Heat other half of the butter in the same pan and sauté cauliflower rice and hemp hearts in it for 2-3 minutes, over medium heat.

3.　　Add in the remaining ingredients and stir well. Reduce the heat to medium-low and cook for a few minutes until the mixture is thick.

4.　　Take off the heat and transfer to serving plates. Put the sautéed mushrooms on top and a little cheddar cheese if you want.

19   Keto Mushroom Sausage Skillet

Servings: 6 | **Time**: 30 mins | **Difficulty**: Easy

Nutrients per serving: Calories: 364 kcal | Fat: 29.3g | Carbohydrates: 4.3g | Protein: 20.1g

Ingredients

2 Tbsps. Olive Oil

2 Cups Pork Sausage

2 Cups Cremini Mushroom, Sliced

1 Cup Mozzarella Cheese, Grated

2 Green Onions, For Garnish

Method

1.   Preheat the broiler in the oven.

2.   Heat 1 tbsp. olive oil in a skillet over medium heat and brown the sausages in it. Take out once done and let cool. Chop them into small pieces.

3.   Heat 1 tbsp. olive oil in the same skillet and sauté the sliced mushrooms in it until become golden brown.

4.   Add in the chopped pork sausage and mozzarella cheese.

5.	Put the skillet in the preheated broiler and cook until the cheese melts.

6.	Take out of the oven and top with green onions.

20 Keto Lemon Donut Holes

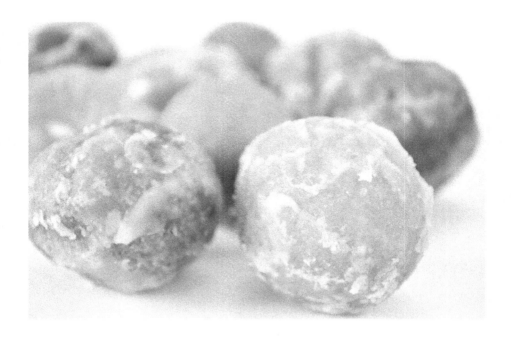

Servings: 10 | **Time:** 15 mins | **Difficulty:** Easy

Nutrients per serving: Calories: 91 kcal | Fat: 8.3g | Carbohydrates: 1.4g | Protein: 2.4g

Ingredients

For Donut Holes:

1/2 Tsp. Vanilla Extract

Wedges of 1/2 Lemon, Seeded

3 Tbsps. Stevia/Erythritol Blend 2 Tbsps. Avocado Oil

1/8 Tsp. Salt

1 Tbsp. Water

1 Cup Almond Flour

For Lemon Glaze:

2 Tsps. Lemon Juice

4 Tbsps. Stevia/Erythritol Blend, Powdered

Method

1.   Preheat the oven to 350 degrees F.

2.   Combine all the donut hole ingredients in a blender and blend well until a thick dough is formed.

3.   Put spoonful of this dough on a lined baking sheet and smooth out in a ball shape using hands.

4.   Put in the preheated oven and bake for 10-12 minutes.

5.   Combine all the glaze ingredients in a bowl and mix well.

6.   Once the donuts are done, take out of the oven and let cool.

7.   Top the donut holes with lemon glaze and serve.

21   Keto Eggs Benedict

Servings: 2 | **Time**: 25 mins | **Difficulty:** Easy

 Nutrients per serving: Calories: 781 kcal | Fat: 60.9g | Carbohydrates: 5.9g | Protein: 50g

Ingredients

Hollandaise Sauce:

1 Tsp. Lemon Juice

Salt, To Taste

2 Egg Yolks

Paprika, To Taste

2 Tbsps. Butter, Melted

2 Tsps. Butter

90 Second Keto Mug Bread For 20 Servings:

1 Tbsp. White Vinegar

4 Eggs

1 Tbsp. Chives, Chopped

4 Canadian Bacon Slices

Salt, To Taste

Method

1.   Cook the keto mug bread according to package instructions, slice it and set aside.

2.   Take a metal bowl and whisk the egg yolks and lemon juice in it, until combined.

3.   Fill half a pot with water and boil over medium heat. Once boiled, lower the heat, and put the metal bowl in it as a double boiler.

4.   Once the yolk mixture heats up, pour the melted butter in it slowly and keep stirring to mix it well with the yolks over low heat.

5.   Do not let the yolks scramble and take the pot out once a thick mixture is formed. Add in the salt and pepper in it and mix well. Set the hollandaise aside.

6.   To prepare the poached eggs, fill a pot with 3-4 inches of water and boil it over medium-high heat. Once it starts boiling, lower the heat and put salt and vinegar in the simmering water.

7.   Crack an egg in a bowl, keeping its yolk intact. Stir the simmering water with a spoon in circular manner to create a whirlpool and slowly pour the egg into the water.

8.   Allow the egg to cook for 2 to 3 minutes, then take it out with a slotted spoon and gently put on a plate with paper towels.

9.   Repeat the process with the rest of the eggs.

10.   Sauté the Canadian bacon slices in a pan until become crispy.

11.   Take a slice of mug bread, put the bacon on it and top bacon with poached egg. Sprinkle some salt and pepper on it if you want. Assemble the egg benedicts like this with other slices too.

12. Top the benedict eggs with a spoonful of hollandaise mixture and chopped chives.

22   Huevos Rancheros

Servings: 4 | **Time**: 25 mins | **Difficulty**: Easy

Nutrients per serving (1 tostada): Calories: 457 kcal | Fat: 37.33g | Carbohydrates: 6.88g | Protein: 20.7g

Ingredients

Chipotle Salsa:

1 Tbsp. Chipotle Peppers In Adobo Sauce

Salt, To Taste

1/2 Cup Tomato Sauce (Low-Carb)

2 Tbsps. Coconut Oil

2 Tsps. Oregano, Dried

Black Pepper, To Taste

2 Tsps. Red Pepper Flakes, Crushed

2 Tsps. Garlic, Fresh & Minced

1/2 Shallot, Diced Finely

Egg Tortilla:

4 Lime Wedges

4 Eggs

1 Avocado, Sliced

1/4 Cup Cilantro, Fresh & Chopped

2 Cups Cheese Blend, Shredded (Mexican-Style)

Method

1.   Heat coconut oil in a skillet over medium heat and sauté crushed red pepper flakes in it for aa minute and take off the heat. Let it rest for some time, strain the oil and get rid of the flakes.

2.   Heat 3/4 of the drained chili oil in the skillet again and sauté the shallots and onion in it until they become fragrant. Add in the tomato sauce, chipotle chili, and oregano and cook them until the sauce thickens. Remove off the heat and set the chili salsa aside.

3.   Add the 1/4 drained chili oil on a non-stick pan and spread the cheese all over the pan, making a layer at the bottom. Cook it over medium-low heat and once it starts to melt, crack the eggs on the top and cover the pan.

4.   Cook at the low heat until the egg whites are cooked through. Increase the heat and let the cheese get crispy and golden. Take the egg tortilla out of the pan on a plate.

5.   Repeat this process to make similar egg tortillas.

6.   Put a spoonful of chili salsa on top of egg tortillas and sprinkle with cilantro. Put lime wedges and avocado slices on the plate too while serving.

23 Keto Breakfast Enchiladas

Servings: 4 | **Time:** 55 mins | **Difficulty**: Easy

Nutrients per serving: Calories: 524.4 kcal | Fat: 42.55g | Carbohydrates: 6.08g | Protein: 27.3g

Ingredients

Tortillas

1/2 Tsp. Chili Powder

6 Eggs

1/4 Tsp. Black Pepper

1/4 Cup Heavy Whipping Cream

1/2 Tsp. Garlic Powder

1/2 Tsp. Salt

1/2 Tsp. Coconut Oil Enchiladas

1 & 1/2 Cups Cheddar Cheese, Shredded

3/4 Cup Enchilada Sauce

1 Cup Sausage, Ground and Cooked

Method

1.   Preheat the oven to 400 degrees F.

2.   Combine all the tortilla ingredients in a bowl and whisk well until become smooth.

3.   Heat coconut oil in a skillet, pour 1/4 cup of the batter in it and cover it.

4.   Cook for 3 to 5 minutes until the eggs are cooked completely.

5.   Repeat this process to make more tortillas with the remaining batter.

6.   Take a tortilla and put a spoonful cooked sausage and cheese on it. Roll the tortilla and set in a casserole dish. Repeat this with all other tortillas.

7.   Top them with enchilada sauce and extra cheese.

8.   Put the casserole dish in the preheated oven and bake for 15 minutes or until the cheese has melted and become golden.

24   Keto Southern Shakshuka

Servings: 6 eggs and sauce | **Time:** 30 mins | **Difficulty:** Easy

Nutrients per serving (1 egg and sauce): Calories: 291.45 kcal | Fat: 19.14g | Carbohydrates: 11.94g | Protein: 15.17g

Ingredients

1.   1/4 Cup Olive Oil

2.   14 Garlic Cloves, Minced

3.   1/2 Cup Goat Cheese, Crumbled

4.   1 Onion, Diced

5.   6 Eggs

6.   3 Cups Collard Greens, Chopped

7.   1 Jalapeño, Chopped

8.   1/2 Green Bell Pepper, Diced

9.   3 & 1/2 Cup Tomatoes, Crushed

10.   1 Tbsp. Paprika Powder

11.   Salt, To Taste

12.   1/2 Tsp. Red Pepper Flakes

13.   Black Pepper, To Taste

Method

1.   Preheat the oven to 425 degrees F.

2.   Heat the olive oil in an oven-safe skillet over medium-high heat and put all the ingredients in it except eggs.

3.   Sauté it well until everything is cooked through. Take off the heat.

4.   Make wells or holes in the sauce with a spoon and put an egg into each well or hole.

5.   Put the skillet in the preheated oven and bake for 5 minutes or until the egg whites are cooked.

6.   Take out and serve with the crumbled goat cheese on top.

25   Keto Chicken and Waffle Sandwiches

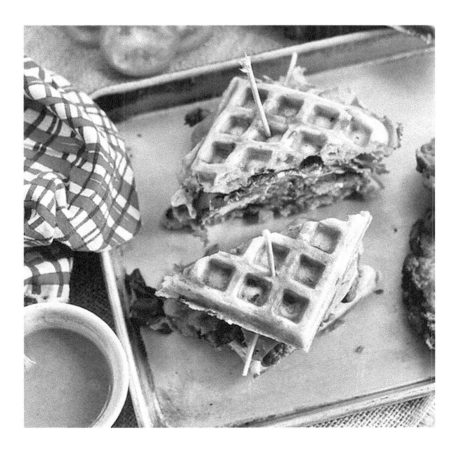

Servings: 4 | **Time:** 25 mins | **Difficulty:** Easy

Nutrients per serving: Calories: 452.9 kcal | Fat: 31.68g | Carbohydrates: 5.1g | Protein: 33.73g

Ingredients

Chicken:

1.   Olive Oil, For Frying

2.   1 Cup Buttermilk

3.   Black Pepper, To Taste

4.   1/3 Cup Almond Flour

5.   Salt, To Taste

6.   1 Tsp. Paprika

7.   2 Chicken Breasts, Halved Lengthwise

8.   1/4 Tsp. Cayenne Powder

9.   1 Egg

10.   Sugar-Free Syrup (Optional)

11.   Bacon (Optional)

12.   Pickles (Optional)

13.   Mustard (Optional)

Waffles:

1. 1/4 Cup Milk

2.   2 Tbsps. Butter, Melted

3.   1 Tbsp. Erythritol

4.   1/2 Tsp. Salt

5.   3 Eggs (Whites & Yolks Separated)

6.   1 Tsp. Vanilla

7.   1 Cup Almond Flour

Method

1.   Preheat the oven at 350 degrees F.

2.   Cut each chicken breasts halve into four strips and soak the strips in buttermilk overnight. Take the chicken strips out of the buttermilk the next day and season with cayenne powder, salt, paprika powder, and black pepper.

3.   Beat the egg in a bowl and set aside.

4.   Whisk the almond flour, some salt and pepper in another bowl and set aside.

5.   Coat the chicken strips first in the egg, then the flour, again in the egg, and lastly the almond flour to make two layers of each.

6.   Heat some olive oil in a skillet and fry the chicken strips in it on both sides until golden brown. Take out and put on a lined baking sheet.

7.   Cover the baking sheet with aluminum foil and put in the preheated oven. Bake for 15 minutes or until cooked through.

8.   Preheat the waffle iron.

9.   Combine the melted butter, egg yolks, vanilla, milk, erythritol, almond flour and salt in a bowl and whisk well until smooth batter is formed.

10.   Take the egg whites in a bowl and whisk them well until they become creamy and fluffy. Add it in the batter.

11.   Spray the waffle iron with a cooking oil spray and pour the batter in it. Cook the waffles for good 5 minutes or until become golden brown.

12.   Sandwich the chicken between the waffles. You can add the bacon and mustard in it if you want and top with maple syrup, if desired.

26 Keto Pepperoni Pizza Quiche

Servings: 8 | **Time:** 55 mins | **Difficulty:** Easy

Nutrients per serving: Calories: 416.66kcal | Fat: 38.43g | Carbohydrates: 4.41g | Protein: 14.29g

Ingredients

The Pie Crust:

6 Tbsps. Butter, Diced (Cold)

1 & 1/2 Cups Almond Flour

1 Egg, Beaten

1 Tsp. Xanthan Gum

1/4 Cup Coconut Flour

1 Tsp. Vinegar

1 Tsp. Salt Quiche

Filling:

6 Eggs

1/4 Tsp. Red Pepper Flakes

1 Cup Mozzarella Cheese, Shredded

1/2 Tsp. Italian Seasoning

Salt, To Taste

15 Pepperoni Slices

Black Pepper, To Taste

1 Cup Heavy Cream

Method

1.   Preheat the oven to 350F.

2.   Combine the coconut flour, xanthan gum, almond flour, vinegar, salt, egg, and butter in a blender and blend until a smooth dough is formed. Take out the dough and cover the dough with plastic wrap. Chill it for 45-60 minutes.

3.   Roll the dough into a 10-inch pie crust. Put in a lined pie plate.

4.   Put half of the mozzarella cheese and pepperoni inside the pie crust.

5.   Combine the eggs, Italian seasoning, heavy cream, salt, red pepper flakes, and black pepper in a bowl and whisk well.

6.   Pour the eggs into the pie crust and sprinkle the remaining cheese and pepperoni on top.

7.   Cover the pie plate with aluminum foil and put in the preheated oven. Bake for about 35-45 minutes.

8.   Take off the foil and bake again until the eggs are fully set, for about 15 minutes.

27   Keto Blueberry Pancake Bites

Servings: 6 | **Time:** 35 mins | **Difficulty:** Easy

Nutrients per serving: Calories: 174.77 kcal | Fat: 13.27g| Carbohydrates: 7.07g | Protein: 6.52g

Ingredients

1/4 Cup Butter, Melted

1/2 Cup Blueberries, Frozen

4 Eggs

1/3 Cup Water

1/2 Cup Coconut Flour

1/4 Tsp. Cinnamon

1/4 Cup Erythritol

1 Tsp. Baking Powder

1/2 Tsp. Vanilla Extract

1/2 Tsp. Salt

Method

1.   Preheat the oven to 325 degrees F.

2.   Combine the eggs, erythritol, coconut flour, baking powder, butter, vanilla extract, salt, and cinnamon in a blender and blend well until smooth. Let it sit for a few minutes. If the batter is very thick, add in the water and blend again.

3.   Pour the batter into a greased muffin tin and put the blueberries on top and press some inside the batter.

4.   Put the muffin tin in the preheated oven and bake for 25 minutes or until the cake bites cooked thoroughly.

28   Gooey Keto Cinnamon Rolls

Servings: 9 | **Time:** 55 mins | **Difficulty:** Easy

Nutrients per serving: Calories: 386.73 kcal | Fat: 31.55g | Carbohydrates: 6.82g | Protein: 16.62g

Ingredients

Cinnamon Rolls:

3 Eggs

6 Tbsps. Golden Flaxseed, Ground

1/4 Cup Sour Cream

5 Tbsps. Erythritol

2 & 1/4 Tsps. Baking Powder

3 Tbsps. Water (Lukewarm)

1 & 1/2 Tbsps. Butter, Unsalted & Melted

5 Tbsps. Whey Protein Isolate

1/8 Tsp. Ginger, Ground

2 & 1/4 Cups Almond Flour

1 Tbsp. Yeast (Active Dry)

1 Tbsp. Maple Syrup

1 Tbsp. Apple Cider Vinegar

2 & 1/4 Tsps. Xanthan Gum

1 & 1/2 Tsp. Kosher Salt

Cinnamon Filling:

2 Tbsps. Cinnamon, Ground

6 Tbsps. Erythritol

3 Tbsps. Butter, Softened

Heavy Cream, To Taste

Glaze:

3 Tbsps. Butter, Unsalted

1 Tsp. Vanilla Extract

1/3 Cup Cream Cheese

Salt, To Taste

3-6 Tbsps. Erythritol, Powdered

Method

1.	Line a baking sheet with parchment paper.

2.	Combine the sour cream, maple syrup, active dry yeast, and warm water in a bowl and mix them well. Cover the bowl, set it aside for 10 minutes to activate the yeast.

3.   Meanwhile, combine the almond flour, whey protein powder, flaxseed meal, baking powder, erythritol, xanthan gum, and salt in another bowl and mix them well.

4.   Once the yeast has been activated – the foam of bubbles is formed at the surface, add in the melted butter eggs, and apple cider vinegar. Whisk them well and put the flour mixture in it too.

5.   Mix the batter well to make it smooth, without any lumps, and slowly a thick dough is formed. Put the dough on a large piece of cling film laid out, knead it into a ball and divide the dough ball into 3 parts. Wet your hands with a mixture of oil and water while handling the dough.

6.   Take one part of the dough and roll/spread it into a rectangle, brush it with melted butter and scatter the erythritol and cinnamon powder on it. Make a roll out of the rectangle and seal it with the help of cling film.

7.   Cut the roll into three mini rolls, take them off the cling film, flatten them with your hands and put on a lined baking pan. Repeat this process with the other two parts of the dough.

8.   With a kitchen towel, cover the pan and set the pan aside in a warm place for an hour, to let the dough rise.

9.   Meanwhile, preheat the oven to 400 degrees F and whisk the glaze ingredients well to make a thick cream.

10.   Once the dough is double in size, put the pan in the preheated oven for about 20-25 minutes, until they become golden brown. Check in between and do not let them brown too much.

11.   Once done, take out of the oven and glaze them before serving. Serve warm.

29 Berry Coconut Oatmeal

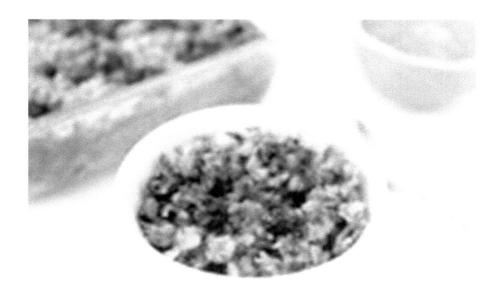

Servings: 1 | **Time:** 8 mins | **Difficulty**: Easy

Nutrients per serving: Calories: 445 kcal | Fat: 38.16g | Carbohydrates: 6.34g | Protein: 10.45g

Ingredients

1/4 Cup Mixed Berries

1/2 Cup Almond Milk

1 Tbsp. Almond Meal

2 Tbsps. Flaxseed, Ground

1 Tsp. Pumpkin Seeds, Dried

1 Tbsp. Coconut, Dried

1/2 Tsp. Cinnamon

1/3 Cup Coconut Milk

1/2 Tsp. Vanilla Powder

Method

1.   Combine all the ingredients in a saucepan, except berries and pumpkin seeds. Heat them over medium flame, with continuous stirring until it thickens and looks like an oatmeal.

2.   Transfer into a bowl and put pumpkin seeds and mixed berries on top.

30 Keto Breakfast Bowl

Servings: 4 | **Time:** 25 mins | **Difficulty:** Easy

Nutrients per serving: Calories: 887.68 kcal | Fat: 75.4g | Carbohydrates: 8.2g | Protein: 40.95g

Ingredients

4 Eggs

1 Cup Coconut Oil

2 Cups Beef Sirloin

6 Garlic Cloves, Minced

2 Cups Cauliflower Rice

1 Tbsp. Erythritol, Granulated

1/8 Cup Calamansi Juice

3 Tsps. Garlic Powder

1/4 Cup Soy Sauce

Salt, To Taste

Black Pepper, To Taste

Method

1.   Take a bowl and put the erythritol, calamansi juice, soy sauce, salt, half the garlic powder and black pepper in it. Mix well until dissolved.

2.   Pour it over the beef in a Ziploc bag and put in the refrigerator overnight.

3.   In the morning, heat one tsp. of coconut oil in a frying pan and sauté the marinated beef in it until cooked through.

4.   Take out and let cool. Then cut into thin strips.

5.   Heat the rest of the coconut oil in the same pan and sauté the garlic in it until fragrant.

6.   Stir in the cauliflower rice and stir well until become soft and dry, sprinkle the other half of the garlic powder, salt, and pepper on it. Stir for a while and take out.

7.   Fry the eggs in the pan, as you like them and serve with cauliflower rice and beef strips.

31　Asparagus and Gruyere Keto Quiche

Servings: 6 | **Time**: 1 hr. 30 mins | **Difficulty:** Easy

Nutrients per serving: Calories: 520 kcal | Fat: 46.39g | Carbohydrates: 4.82g | Protein: 21.17g

Ingredients

Crust:

1/4 Cup Butter, Melted

1 Cup Almond Flour

1/2 Tsp. Xanthan Gum

1 Egg White

1/2 Cup Gruyere, Grated

2 Tbsps. Coconut Flour

2/3 Cup Gruyere. Cubed

Filling:

1 Egg Yolk

1 Shallot, Sliced

1 Tsp. Salt

4 Eggs

1 Cup Heavy Cream

Oil, To Taste

Method

1.   Preheat the oven to 350 degrees F.

2.   Combine all the crust ingredients in a bowl and whisk or beat well to make a smooth dough.

3.   Knead the dough into a ball and refrigerate it for 30 minutes.

4.   Take out the dough and press in a lined pie pan to spread till the edges.

5.   Put in the preheated oven to bake for 10 minutes, then take out and let cool.

6.   Whisk the egg yolk with heavy cream, eggs, and salt to form a creamy mixture.

7.   Heat oil in a pan and sauté the shallot and asparagus in it until they become tender. Set aside.

8.   For the assembly, first put the gruyere in the base of the quiche crust, then put the cheese, onion and asparagus on its top, then our in the eggs mixture.

9.   Bake for 45-60 minutes or until the surface is golden brown and the eggs are completely cooked.

32 Keto Lemon Sugar Poppy Seed Scones

Servings: 8 | **Time:** 45 mins | **Difficulty**: Easy

Nutrients per serving: Calories: 206.81 kcal | Fat: 18.5g | Carbohydrates: 3.53g | Protein: 6.6g

Ingredients

4 Tbsps. Butter

1 & 1/2 Cups Almond Flour

1/2 Tsp. Baking Powder

1 Tbsp. Lemon Juice

2 Tbsps. Coconut Flour

1/4 Tsp. Baking Soda

1/4 Cup + 2 Tbsps. Erythritol

1 Tbsp. Poppy Seeds

1 Tbsp. Lemon Zest

2 Eggs

1 Tbsp. Psyllium Husk Fiber

Method

1.   Preheat the oven to 350 degrees F.

2.   Combine all the ingredients in a bowl, except the lemon zest and 2 tbsps. erythritol. Whisk them well to make a smooth dough, without lumps.

3.   Combine the lemon zest and 2 tbsps. of erythritol in a bowl and mix well. Set aside to let dry.

4.   Knead the dough into a ball, then roll I on a clean surface to form a thick dough sheet and cut eight triangles out of it.

5.   Put the dough triangles on a lined baking sheet and bake in the preheated oven for 20 minutes.

6.   Take out of the oven, sprinkle with lemon sugar, and bake for another 10 minutes.

33   Eggs Benedict Casserole

Servings: 8 | **Time:** 45 mins | **Difficulty:** Medium

Nutrients per serving: Calories: 483 kcal | Fat: 33.41g | Carbohydrates: 2.78g | Protein: 18.54g

Ingredients

2 Tbsps. White Vinegar

1/4 Cup Heavy Whipping Cream

Lemon Juice, To Taste

1 Cup Butter, Unsalted & Melted

6 Egg Yolks

1/4 Tsp. Peppercorns, Crushed

Salt, To Taste

1 Tbsp. Water

2 & 1/2 Cups Eggplant, Peeled & Diced

2 Cups Ham, Cooked & Diced

12 Eggs

Black Pepper, To Taste

Method

1.   Preheat the oven to 375 degrees F.

2.   Take a greased casserole dish and spread the diced eggplant in the bottom and make a layer of ham on top of it.

3.   Whisk the eggs, cream, salt, and pepper in a bowl and pour over the ham layer and stir to let it reach to the bottom.

4.   Cover the casserole dish with a foil and put in the preheated oven for 30 minutes.

5.   Take out of the oven and remove the foil. Bake it again for 20-30 minutes or until the egg is completely cooked.

6.   Add vinegar and crushed peppercorns in a preheated skillet and stir until the vinegar evaporates, add the water and transfer this to a metal bowl.

7.   Boil water in a pan, lower the heat to let it simmer and put the metal bowl in it. Add the egg yolks into the metal bowl and whisk well. Do not let the yolk scramble and whisk at low heat until the yolks thicken.

8.   Take the bowl out of the water pot and slowly add the clear melted butter in it while whisking the yolks continuously.

9.   Add lemon and salt to taste and 2-3 Tbsps. of water if the consistency of the sauce is very thick. Do not dilute it out too much though.

10.   Once the casserole is cooked, pour the sauce over it and serve hot.

34   Bacon Kale and Tomato Frittata

Servings: 6 | **Time**: 35 mins | **Difficulty**: Easy

Nutrients per serving: Calories: 292.5 kcal | Fat: 24.88g | Carbohydrates: 1.61g | Protein: 13.77g

Ingredients

7 Eggs

1 Tbsp. Mayonnaise

7 Bacon Strips

1/2 Cup Parmesan Cheese, Shredded

2 Parsley Sprigs, Chopped

1/4 Cup Heavy Whipping Cream

1 Cup Kale, Destemmed & Chopped

5 Cherry Tomatoes, Sliced

Method

1.   Preheat the oven to 400 degrees F.

2.   Combine the eggs with whipping cream, mayonnaise, and cheese in a bowl and whisk well until combined. Set aside.

3.   Sauté the bacon strips in a non-stick pan over medium-low flame until they become crispy. Take out once done and put on a paper towel. Let cool and then crumble the strips.

4.   Sauté the kale in the same pan until it becomes tender and put the 3/4 of the crumbled bacon back in the pan. Stir well.

5.   Pour in the egg mixture and stir to combine, once the eggs are about to set, add in the 3/4 of the tomato slices and cook for another minute.

6.   Then remove the skillet off the heat and put the frittata in preheated oven for 5-10 minutes or until cooked thoroughly.

7.   Sprinkle with crumbled bacon and tomato slices and parsley on top.

35 Caprese Egg Casserole

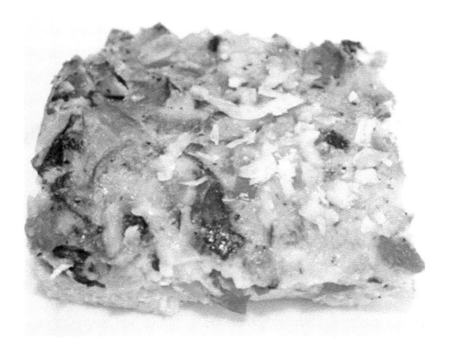

Servings: 2 | **Time**: 45 mins | **Difficulty**: Easy

Nutrients per serving: Calories: 151 kcal | Fat: 11.38g | Carbohydrates: 1.68g | Protein: 9.8g

Ingredients

8 Eggs

1/2 Cup Mozzarella Balls, Fresh

Black Pepper, To Taste

2 Tbsps. Olive Oil

Salt, To Taste

1 Tbsp. Basil, Fresh & Chopped

2 Cups Cherry Tomatoes, Halved

Method

1.   Preheat the oven to 350 degrees F.

2.   Heat the olive oil in a skillet and sauté the halved tomatoes in it util they have softened, and do not dry them out. Set aside to let cool.

3.   Whisk the eggs with chopped basil, salt, and pepper in a bowl until smooth.

4.   Brush a casserole dish with some oil or butter and pour the eggs mixture in it. Add the cooked tomatoes and mozzarella balls on top.

5.   Bake for 25-30 minutes in the preheated oven, or until the eggs are cooked through.

36 Keto Sausage Gravy and Biscuit Bake

Servings: 6 | **Time:** 35 mins | **Difficulty**: Easy

Nutrients per serving: Calories: 374.67 kcal | Fat: 33.21g | Carbohydrates: 4.75g | Protein: 14.48g

Ingredients

Biscuits:

1/2 Tsp. Xanthan Gum

1 Cup Almond Flour

2 Egg Whites

2 Tbsps. Butter, Cold & Grated

1 Tsp. Baking Powder

Sausage Gravy:

3/4 Cup Pork Sausage, Ground

1/2 Tsp. Onion Powder

1/2 Cup Half And Half

1 Tsp. Black Pepper

1 Tsp. Xanthan Gum

1/4 Tsp. Salt

1 & 1/2 Cups Chicken Broth

Method

1.   Preheat the oven to 375 degrees F.

2.   Put all the biscuit ingredients in a bowl and mix well until combined and refrigerate it for some time.

3.   Meanwhile, brown the ground pork in a skillet over medium heat until cooked through. Take out and set aside.

4.   Sauté the xanthan gum in the same skillet in the pork fat for 1 minute or until become light brown, over medium-low heat.

5.   Stir in the chicken stock, black pepper, onion powder, and salt. Let the gravy simmer for about 5 minutes then add half and half and mix well.

6.   Let it simmer for another 3 minutes or until the gravy becomes thick and creamy.

7.   Add the pork in it as well and stir to heat up. Take off the heat.

8.   Grease a casserole dish with oil or butter and pour the sausage gravy in it.

9.   Spread the biscuit mixture on the top, making an even layer.

10.   Put the casserole dish in the preheated oven and bake for 18-20 minutes, until the biscuit mixture is cooked through.

37 Mini Pizza Egg Bakes

Servings: 1 | **Time:** 15 mins | **Difficulty:** Easy

Nutrients per serving (2 Mini Pizza): Calories: 333 kcal | Fat: 22.66g | Carbohydrates: 4.28g | Protein: 25.59g

Ingredients

1 Tbsp. Red Bell Pepper, Diced

3 Eggs, Egg & Yolks Separated

2 Black Olives, Sliced

4 Tbsps. Mozzarella Cheese, Shredded

4 Large Mild Pepper Rings

1 Tbsp. Tomato Sauce

1 Tsps. Italian Herb Blend

Method

1.   Whisk the egg whites slightly in an oven safe dish and put the 1 tbsp. of mozzarella cheese and beaten yolks in it and stir slightly.

2.   Microwave it for one and a half minute and let cool for some time.

3.   Put the mild pepper rings on it and spread tomato sauce on the top.

4.   Top it with the diced bell pepper, and olives.

5.   Sprinkle the shredded cheese on it and microwave for a minute or until the cheese melts and become golden.

6.   Serve hot!

38 Instant Pot Crustless Quiche Lorraine

Servings: 4 | **Time:** 45 mins | **Difficulty**: Easy

Nutrients per serving: Calories: 572.5 kcal | Fat: 52.54g | Carbohydrates: 3.46g | Protein: 22.03g | Fiber: 0.03g

Ingredients

1 & 1/3 Cups Swiss Cheese, Shredded

1/4 Tsp. Nutmeg

4 Eggs

1 & 1/2 Cups Heavy Whipping Cream

Pepper, To Taste

8 Bacon Slices, Chopped

1/4 Tsp. Salt

Method

1.   Sauté the bacon slices in a pan until become crispy. Put on the paper towel and set aside.

2.   Combine the eggs, nutmeg, heavy whipping cream, salt, and pepper in a bowl and whisk well until smooth.

3.   Brush a cake pan with butter or oil and spread 1 cup cheese at the bottom of pan. Pour in the creamy egg mixture on top. Cover the pan with foil.

4.   Pour the water in an Instant Pot and put the steam rack inside it. Put the cake pan on the rack carefully and close the Instant Pot lid.

5.   Set high pressure setting, and 25 minutes timer.

6.   Once done, take the cake pan out carefully and top with remaining 1/3 cup shredded cheese.

7.   Broil it for 5-10 minutes or until the cheese becomes golden and let cool.

8.   Serve by flipping out on a serving plate.

39 Vegetarian Three Cheese Quiche Stuffed Peppers

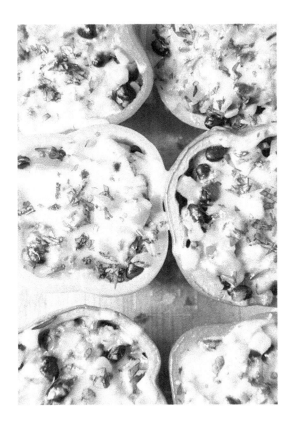

Servings: 4 | **Time**: 55 mins | **Difficulty**: Easy

Nutrients per serving: Calories: 245.5 kcal | Fat: 16.28g | Carbohydrates: 5.97g | Protein: 17.84g | Fiber: 1.13g

Ingredients

1/2 Cup Parmesan Cheese, Grated

4 Eggs

1/4 Cup Baby Spinach Leaves

1/2 Cup Mozzarella Cheese, Shredded

1 Tsp. Garlic Powder

2 Bell Peppers, Deseeded and Halved Lengthwise

1/2 Cup Ricotta Cheese

2 Tbsps. Parmesan Cheese, For Garnishing

1/4 Tsp. Parsley, Dried

Method

1.   Preheat the oven to 375 degrees F.

2.   Put the eggs, cheeses, garlic powder, and parsley in a food processor and blend until combined. Take out and stir in the spinach leaves.

3.   Put the Bell pepper halves on a lined baking sheet and pour the egg and cream mixture in each and cover with foil.

4.   Put in the preheated oven and bake for 35-45 minutes or until the egg is set.

5.   Take out, remove the foil, and sprinkle the 2 Tbsps. Parmesan cheese on top.

6.   Broil for 3-5 minutes or until the cheese melts and becomes golden.

40   No-tatoes Bubble 'n' Squeak

Servings: 3 | **Time:** 35 mins | **Difficulty:** Easy

Nutrients per serving: Calories: 332.67 kcal | Fat: 28.11g | Carbohydrates: 8.6g | Protein: 10.65g | Fiber: 3.23g

Ingredients

2 Tbsps. Butter

Black Pepper, To Taste

Florets Of 1/2 Cauliflower

 Salt, To Taste

2 Tbsps. Heavy Whipping Cream

1/4 Cup Leek, Sliced

2 Tbsps. Duck Fat

1/4 Cup Parmesan Cheese, Grated

1/4 Cup Brussels Sprouts, Chopped

3 Bacon Slices, Diced

1/4 Cup Mozzarella Cheese, Grated

1/4 Onion, Diced

1 Green Onion Stalk, Sliced

1 Tsp. Garlic, Minced

Method

1.   Combine 1 tbsp. butter, cauliflower florets, cream, salt and pepper in a bowl, microwave for 4 minutes on high, and stir well.

2.   Microwave for another 4 minutes, take out and blend with an immersion blender until it becomes smooth.

3.   Add in the mozzarella cheese and stir to melt in the hot mixture. Set aside.

4.   Sauté the chopped bacon in a pan until becomes crispy and put on a paper towel.

5.   Put the remaining butter in the same pan and sauté the garlic in it over medium heat until fragrant.

6.   Add in the onion and sauté it until becomes translucent and then put brussels sprouts and leeks in it. Cook them for about 5-10 minutes or until become soft.

7.   Add in the green onions and cook for another minute. Then take the pan off the heat and let cool.

8.   Combine the veggies with the bacon and mashed cauliflower.

9.   Heat the duck fat in a pan over medium heat and add the mixture in it once the duck fat is melted, top with Parmesan cheese and stir for a while until the cheese melts. Remove from heat.

10.   Transfer on the serving plates and enjoy.

41 **Bacon Breakfast Bagels**

Servings: 3 | **Time:** 25 mins | **Difficulty**: Easy

Nutrients per serving: Calories: 605.67 kcal | Fat: 50.29g | Carbohydrates: 5.76g | Protein: 30.13g | Fiber: 3.87g

Ingredients

1 Egg

2 Tbsps. Cream Cheese

1 Tsp. Xanthan Gum

1 & 1/2 Cups Mozzarella Cheese, Grated

3/4 Cup Almond Flour

6 Bacon Slices, Grilled & Chopped

2 Tbsps. Cream Cheese

2 Tbsps. Pesto

1 Cup Arugula Leaves

Sesame Seeds, To Taste

1 Tbsp. Butter, Melted

Method

1.   Preheat the oven to 390 degrees F.

2.   Combine the mozzarella cream cheese and melt in the oven, add in the almond flour and xanthan gum, and mix well to form a smooth dough.

3.   Knead the dough into a ball, microwave it for 10 seconds if becomes hard.

4.   Divide the dough into 3 parts and roll each part to form three circles.

5.   Line a baking dish with parchment paper and put the three dough circles on it, cut a hollow circle within each using a cookie cutter or jar cap.

6.   Brush the bagels top with melted butter and sprinkle sesame seeds on it.

7.   Put the baking sheet in the preheated oven for about 18 minutes or until bagels become golden brown. Take out once done and let cool.

8.   Cut the bagels in half, spread cream cheese on them, pour the pesto over it, sprinkle with arugula leaves and chopped bacon.

42   Spinach, Herb & Feta Wrap

Servings: 2 | **Time:** 20 mins | **Difficulty:** Easy

Nutrients per serving: Calories: 361.5 kcal | Fat: 25.27g | Carbohydrates: 4.06g | Protein: 27.55g | Fiber: 0.9g

Ingredients

3 Tomatoes, Sundried & Chopped

1/2 Cup Feta Cheese, Crumbled

2 Cups Spinach Leaves

1/2 Tsp. Salt

5 Eggs

1 Tsp. Sesame Oil

4 Basil Leaves, Chopped

3 Egg Whites

1 Tsp. Olive Oil (Optional)

Method

1.   Combine the eggs, egg whites, sesame oil, and salt in a bowl and whisk well to form a foamy mixture.

2.   Heat a non-stick pan over medium heat, lower the heat, and pour half the mixture in it and spread with back of the spoon.

3.   Cook on both sides and put on a plate once done. Make another wrap similarly.

4.   Sauté the spinach in a pan until it wilts and becomes soft.

5.   On each wrap first put the cooked spinach leaves, then feta cheese and basil leaves. Drizzle some oil too if you want and roll the wrap in parchment paper.

43   Salmon Benny Breakfast Bombs

Servings: 2 | **Time:** 55 mins | **Difficulty:** Easy

Nutrients per serving: Calories: 295 kcal | Fat: 23.53g | Carbohydrates: 0.96g | Protein: 18.25g | Fiber: 0.05g

Ingredients

Breakfast Bombs:

1/2 Tbsp. Butter, Salted

2 Tbsps. Chives, Fresh & Chopped

Salt, To Taste

1/2 Cup Salmon, Smoked & Diced

2 Eggs, Hard Boiled

Black Pepper, To Taste

Hollandaise Sauce:

Salt, To Taste

1/4 Tsp. Dijon Mustard

2 Tsps. Lemon Juice

1 Egg Yolk

2 Tbsps. Butter, Melted

1/2 Tbsp. Water

Method

1.   Boil half the pot full of water over medium heat and then lower the heat to let it simmer.

2.   Take metal bowl and combine the lemon juice, egg yolk, salt, and Dijon mustard in it. Put the bowl in the simmering water and whisk the mixture until smooth.

3.   Once the mixture starts to thicken, add in the melted butter slowly and keep whisking to emulsify the mixture. Once thicken, take the bowl out of the pot. Add a little water if hollandaise sauce seems too thick. Let it cool down.

4.   Mash the boiled eggs in a large bowl really well and add in the smoked salmon, hollandaise sauce, and half the chives in it. Mix well until combined. Do not make it too wet. Limit the sauce.

5.   Divide the mixture into four parts and make four balls out of it.

6.   Coat balls with remaining chives by rolling in them and serve.

44   Ham, Ricotta, and Spinach Casserole

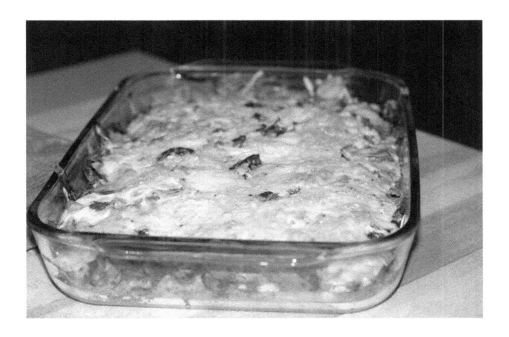

Servings: 2 | **Time:** 40 mins | **Difficulty**: Easy

Nutrients per serving: Calories: 151.8 kcal | Fat: 9.09g | Carbohydrates: 1.35g | Protein: 15.1g | Fiber: 0.41g

Ingredients

1 Cup Spinach, Frozen

1/2 Yellow Onion, Chopped Finely

12 Eggs

1 Cup Ricotta Cheese

1/2 Tbsp. Garlic And Herb Seasoning

2 Cups Ham, Diced

1/4 Tsp. Salt

1/4 Cup Heavy Whipping Cream

Cooking Spray

Method

1.   Preheat the oven to 350 degrees F.

2.   Combine all the ingredients in a bowl and mix well.

3.   Spray a casserole dish with cooking spray and pour in the batter.

4.   Bake in the preheated oven for 30-35 minutes or until cooked thoroughly.

45   Keto Zucchini Bread with Walnuts

Servings: 16 | **Time:** 1 hr. 30 mins | **Difficulty:** Easy

Nutrients per serving: Calories: 200.13 kcal | Fat: 18.83g | Carbohydrates: 2.6g | Protein: 5.59g | Fiber: 2.3g

Ingredients

1/2 Cup Olive Oil

1/4 Tsp. Ginger, Ground

3 Eggs

1/2 Cup Walnuts, Chopped

1 Tsp. Vanilla Extract

1 Cup Zucchini, Grated & Dried

1 Tsp. Cinnamon, Ground

2 & 1/2 Cups Almond Flour

1/2 Tsp. Salt

1 & 1/2 Cups Erythritol

1/2 Tsp. Nutmeg

1 & 1/2 Tsps. Baking Powder

Cooking Spray

Method

1.   Preheat oven to 350 degrees F.

2.   Combine all the ingredients in a bowl and whisk well.

3.   Spray a loaf pan with cooking spray and put the batter in it.

4.   Put in the preheated oven and bake for 60-70 minutes.

46 Lemon Raspberry Sweet Rolls

Servings: 8 | **Time**: 45 mins | **Difficulty:** Easy

Nutrients per serving: Calories: 272.25 kcal | Fat: 23.18g | Carbohydrates: 5.24g | Protein: 10.04g | Fiber: 2.28g

Ingredients

1/2 Cup Cream Cheese

1/2 Cup Raspberries, Frozen

2 Tbsps. Butter, Melted

1 Tsp. Lemon Extract

4 Tbsps. Stevia/Erythritol Blend

1/4 Tsp. Xanthan Gum

1/2 Tsp. Vanilla Extract

1 Tbsp. Water

2 Tsps. Lemon Zest

3 Tsp. Lemon Juice

1 Egg

1 Tsp. Vanilla Extract

1 Cup Almond Flour

2 Cups Mozzarella Cheese

1/4 Tsp. Xanthan Gum

1/4 Cup Stevia Erythritol Blend

1 & 1/4 Tsps. Baking Powder

Method

1.   Combine the softened cream cheese, 2 tbsps. sweetener melted butter, vanilla extract, lemon zest, lemon extract and 1 tsp. of lemon juice in a bowl and whisk well to make a smooth and creamy mixture. Set this lemon cream cheese filling aside.

2.   Heat 2 tbsps. of sweetener, xanthan gum and 2 Tsps. of lemon juice in a saucepan over medium-low heat with constant stirring.

3.   Add in the frozen raspberries and mix well. Once the raspberries become warm, turn off the heat and set this raspberry sauce aside.

4.   Preheat the oven to 350 degrees F.

5.   Combine all the dough ingredients in a metal bowl and mix.

6.   Fill one quarter of a pot with water and boil it over medium heat. Once boiled, lower the heat to let the water simmer, and put the metal bowl on it. Melting the cheese will make the mixing of the dough easier. Whisk the batter well until smooth, then take out of the pot.

7.   Knead the dough well and roll to form a 12x15 inches rectangle.

8.   Spread the lemon cream cheese filling on the dough evenly, and then make layer of raspberry sauce on top, leaving 1-inch dough from a side.

9.   Roll the dough into a log starting at the long side and press to seal at the other side.

10.   With a sharp knife cut the log into 8 pieces, gently and put these pieces on a lined baking sheet.

11.   Put in the oven and bake for 24-26 minutes, or until the rolls become golden brown.

47   Keto Faux Sous Vide Egg Bites

Servings: 16 (8 per flavor) | **Time:** 30 mins | **Difficulty**: Easy

Nutrients per serving: Calories: 140.63 kcal | Fat: 11.05g | Carbohydrates: 0.65g | Protein: 9.19g | Fiber: 0.01g

Ingredients

1 Tsp. Hot Sauce

Salt, To Taste

2 Tbsps. Monterey Jack Cheese, Grated

6 Bacon Strips, Cooked

Black Pepper, To Taste

2 Tbsps. Chives, Chopped

6 Eggs

Additional Seasonings, To Taste

1/4 Cup Gruyere Cheese, Grated

2 Tbsps. Butter

1/4 Cup Cottage Cheese

Method

1.   Combine all the ingredients in a bowl except bacon and whisk well until a smooth mixture is formed.

2.   Take poaching pan and pour water in the bottom. Set the heat to medium-high and in each well of the pan put a slice of bacon at the bottom and spoonful whisked mixture on top.

3.   Once the water of the pan begins to simmer, lower the heat to medium and cover the pan. Cook for 5-7 minutes or until the egg bites are firm from center. Take out.

48   Savory Sage and Cheddar Waffles

Servings: 12 | **Time:** 25 mins | **Difficulty**: Easy

Nutrients per serving: Calories: 195.5 kcal | Fat: 17.47g | Carbohydrates: 3.49g | Protein: 5.49g | Fiber: 5.35g

Ingredients

1 & 1/3 Cup Coconut Flour

1/4 Tsp. Garlic Powder

2 Cups Coconut Milk

1/2 Cup Water

3 Tbsps. Coconut Oil, Melted

3 Tsps. Baking Powder

1 Cup Cheddar Cheese, Shredded

2 Eggs

1 Tsp. Sage, Dried & Ground

1/2 Tsp. Salt

Method

1.   Preheat the waffle iron.

2.   Combine all the ingredients in a bowl and whisk well to form a smooth batter.

3.   Put the batter in the waffle iron in the quantity that fits in it and close it.

4.   Cook until they become golden brown.

5.   Take out and serve with a low carb topping.

49 Keto Lemon Poppyseed Muffins

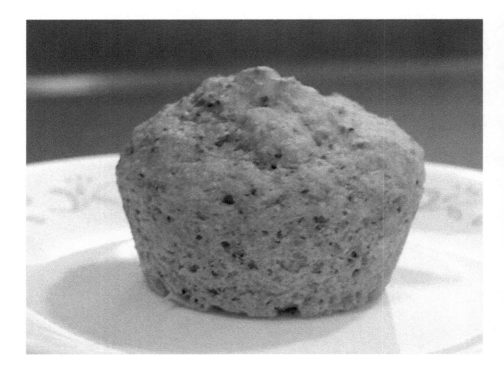

Servings: 12 | **Time:** 45 mins | **Difficulty:** Easy

Nutrients per serving: Calories: 99.89 kcal | Fat: 11.69g | Carbohydrates: 1.73g | Protein: 4.04g | Fiber: 1.65g

Ingredients

1 Tsp. Vanilla Extract

3/4 Cup Almond Flour

3 Eggs

4 Tsps. Lemon Zest

1/4 Cup Heavy Cream

2 Tbsps. Poppy Seeds

1/4 Cup Golden Flaxseed Meal

1/3 Cup Erythritol

1/4 Cup Butter, Melted

3 Tbsps. Lemon Juice

1 Tsp. Baking Powder

25 Drops Liquid Stevia

Method

1.   Preheat the oven to 350 degrees F.

2.   Combine all the ingredients in a bowl and whisk well to form a smooth batter.

3.   Grease a 12-cup muffin tin and put the batter in them equally.

4.   Bake in the preheated oven for 18-20 minutes or until cooked through.

5.   Take out and let cool, then serve.

50 Low Carb Mock McGriddle Casserole

Servings: 8 | **Time**: 1 hr. 15 mins | **Difficulty:** Easy

Nutrients per serving: Calories: 447.63 kcal | Fat: 36.04g | Carbohydrates: 2.87g | Protein: 26.16g | Fiber: 2.3g

Ingredients

6 Tbsps. Maple Syrup

1/2 Tsp. Garlic Powder

1 Cup Almond Flour

Salt, To Taste

1/4 Cup Flaxseed Meal

2 Cups Breakfast Sausage

1/2 Tsp. Onion Powder

10 Eggs

Black Pepper, To Taste

1/2 Cup Cheddar Cheese

4 Tbsps. Butter, Melted

1/4 Tsp. Sage

Method

1.   Pre-heat the oven to 350 degrees F.

2.   Cook the breakfast sausage in a pan over medium heat and break it while cooking.

3.   Combine all the ingredients in a bowl, including the sausage and mix well.

4.   Put the mixture in a lined casserole dish and put in the preheated oven.

5.   Bake for 45-55 minutes until cooked through and golden brown from top.

Lightning Source UK Ltd.
Milton Keynes UK
UKHW021845040521
383144UK00003B/351